Snacks Can Be Nutritious And Good Choices For Kids

• •

Evelyn J. Echols

authorHOUSE®

AuthorHouse™
1663 Liberty Drive
Bloomington, IN 47403
www.authorhouse.com
Phone: 1-800-839-8640

First published by AuthorHouse   11/09/2011

ISBN: 978-1-4685-0059-2 (sc)
ISBN: 978-1-4685-0058-5 (ebk)

Library of Congress Control Number: 2011960534

Printed in the United States of America

Any people depicted in stock imagery provided by Thinkstock are models, and such images are being used for illustrative purposes only.
Certain stock imagery © Thinkstock.

This book is printed on acid-free paper.

Contents

I dedicate this book to my wonderful grandchildren whom have brought so much joy in my life. To Elijah, Erin Grace and Kadrian, have patience with me guys; I'm still a Granny in training having fun.

Granny Gigi ♥

Introduction

A **snack** is a portion of food often smaller than that of a regular meal, that is generally eaten between meals. Getting children to try different foods can be a task especially if you have a choosey or picky eater. Mealtime can be a fun time for your child and for you. Eating the same snack everyday isn't much fun. Letting a child help prepare a variety of meals or snacks makes mealtime family time. Allowing children to set the table is a good example for independence and improvement of hand motor skills. Until a child has a little more practice at setting tables, don't use your best dishes. Try using your favorite disposable dinnerware, cups, napkins, and plastic ware. Young children often make mistakes and accidentally can drop or spill things and be messy eaters. Allow your child to clean up their mistakes and only help them when necessary. Family time is when everyone is seated at the table. Let your child pass a food dish, making sure it's not too hot for them to handle such as gravy and soups. Allow your child to serve themselves and choose how much food they do or do not desire to eat. If they are hungry, a child will normally ask for more. A new food should be accompanied with some of the favorite foods of your child's. At this time, they also can learn their table manners such as, "please pass" or "thank you". During mealtime make sure there are no distractions. Television, radio and playing with video games or hand held games at the table are a few examples. Begin conversation with opening statements such as "How was your day at school?" or "What would you like to do this weekend?" Remember, never force a child to eat or clean their plate. Allow them to respond with "No thank you" if they chose not to eat a certain food. Suppose your child doesn't like a food such as green peas, it's ok. It takes sometimes several serving tries before they are willing to try a bite. The best example of course, will be you, the parent. Be a model for your child. Even if you don't like green peas, never say "yuck". Try saying "I think I will try a bite or two". Serve a variety of foods and talk about the flavor, color, texture or where or how the food is grown. As a project, growing a garden may also help your child to attempt a "No thank you bite" with new foods such as peas. Children will always try a bite of what they help to grow. Whether its mealtime or a project growing a garden, you will establish more bonding and trust with your child as a parent or grandparent. After mealtime is over, let your children clean up their place setting or mess from the table. They can place their dishes in the dishwasher, after the food crapes are in the trash, place the dishes in the sink or counter or just place the disposable dinnerware in the trash. They may need help in the beginning. Remember, young children will make mistakes but "Practice makes perfect" and "Patience is a virtue". Good Luck!

Think Variety

Think variety; choose a snack for each day to create with your child. Remember, this is family time so the more the merrier. It may even be a good idea to invite some of your child's friends once in a while to join in the fun. No one likes to eat along. If your schedule is busy, set aside a time for you and your child. Weekends are a great time! Create an activity to go along with the snack or follow the activities suggested in this book. Remember a parent's attitude can influence a child's willingness to try new foods or do activities. Introduce one new food at a time, given in small qualities. Slowly incorporate the new food into regular mealtime. Record your progress on the food chart.

A Few Facts About Fruits and Vegetables

♥ Fruits and vegetables are naturally sweet, low in sodium, have no cholesterol, low fat, low in calories and provide carbohydrates for energy.

♥ A variety of fruits and vegetables are available year round whether fresh, frozen, dried, and canned and as 100% juice.

♥ Fruits and vegetables can be a good natural source of vitamins, and fiber. It is a good source for a healthy snack and represents 2 of the basic food groups choices for a healthy lifestyle.

Snack Recipes

1. Vegetable Pizza	11. Veggie Dip
2. Hummus	12. Southern Fresh Rhubarb Strawberry Fruit
3. Pineapple Cheesecake	13. Pineapple Sweet Potato
4. Fruit Soda	14. Trail Mix
5. Pineapple Orange Yogurt Pops	15. Strawberry Cream Cheese Gingersnap Sandwich
6. Mix Berry Parfait	16. Cinnamon Spiced Apple Sauce
7. Polar Ice Cubes	17. Peanut Butter Rice Crisp
8. Taco Pizza Bagel	18. Turkey Nachos In a Bag
9. Veggie Croissant	19. Friendship Fruit Salad
10. Caribbean Island Fruit Sorbet	20 Making Papa Bread

Activities

How to Grow a Potato Garden From Sprouted Potatoes	Discussion: Where do vegetables grow? Vine, Under Earth, Tree
Multi Cultures	Picture Book Art
Making A Pineapple	Polar Snowman
Saint Patrick's Day	Making a Cinco De Mayo Kite
Ice Cream Day/Puzzle	Making a Rose Flower
Beach Day	On the Animal Trail
Friends	Johnny Apple Seed

Extras

Food Record	Fiber Rich Foods	Iron Rich Foods	Eight Ways To Move
Child Size Servings	Buying Calendar For Fresh Fruits	Buying Calendar For Fresh Veggies	Truths

RECIPES

Vegetable Pizza

½ cup of each fresh vegetables

chopped onions, green bell pepper slices, celery, cauliflower,
broccoli, carrots, radishes, tomatoes, mushrooms,

1 cup of shredded cheddar cheese

1 cup of shredded Monterey Jack cheese

2 packages of crescent rolls

16 ounce tub of soften cream cheese

aluminum pizza pan

Directions:

Place crescent rolls on large round size aluminum disposable pizza pan. Press together at seams with fingers. Bake at 350 degrees for 8 to 10 minutes. When crust has cooled, begin spreading cream cheese on top of crust generously. Top with sliced vegetables and spread Monterey and Cheddar cheese on top of vegetables. Refrigerate for 2 to 4 hours. Serve in small bite pieces.

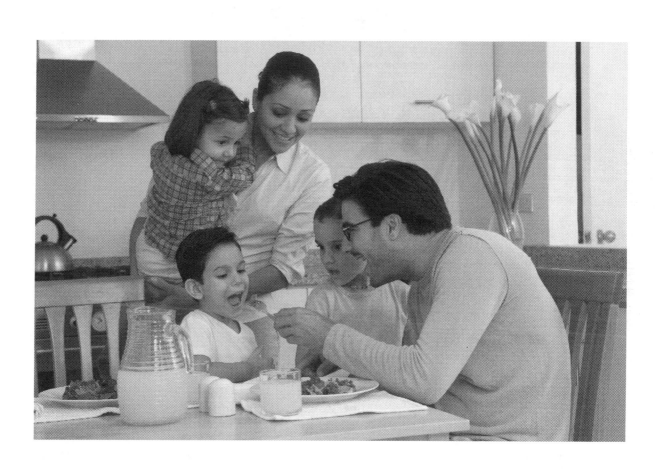

Hummus

1 can of garbanzo beans, drained (reserve liquid)

1/3 cup of tahini

1 tablespoon of olive oil

2 to 4 cloves of garlic, minced

¼ cup of fresh lemon juice (1 to 2 lemons)

2 to 6 tablespoons of liquid from beans

paprika

cumin (optional)

French bread

Directions:

Place beans, Tahini, garlic, lemon juice, olive oil in a food processor or blender. Blend mixture until smooth. Add liquid 1 tablespoon at a time to mixture to your preference of smoothness. Place mixture into a serving bowl and sprinkle paprika on top. If desire you may lightly sprinkle cumin for a stronger flavor. Serve with pita bread, raw vegetables, crackers or toasted French bread slices.

Pineapple Cheesecake

1 cup of graham crackers (crumbs)

2 tablespoons of cornstarch

1 tablespoon of cold water

8 ounce can of crush pineapple (in its own juice)

1 cup of boiling water

¼ cup of sugar

1 ½ pounds of 1% of cottage cheese

2 tablespoons of water

3 ounce package of lemon flavored gelatin

Directions:

Mix graham cracker crumbs and margarine together and place into the bottom of the 8 inch springform pan. Dissolve gelatin in boiling water and let cool to room temperature. Mix cottage cheese, sugar into blender. Slowly add gelatin a little at a time. Blend well. Pour cheese mixture into crust and chill until firm. Dissolve cornstarch in cold water and place into a saucepan. Take pineapple with juice stir into mixture. Bring to a boil stirring until mixture thickens. Cool for 10 to 15minutes. Spread mixture on cheesecake. Place into refrigerator another 15 to 20 minutes for coolness. Enjoy!!

Fruit Soda

Mix together into a pitcher the following juices 8 ounce cans:

Mixture #1

100% cranberry juice

100% apple juice

100% grape juice

100% orange juice

Or

Mixture #2

100% cherry juice

100% apple juice

100% grape juice

Other ingredient: club soda

Directions:

Pour into a glass ½ cup of juice mixture then add ¼ cup of club soda. Note: This is to take the place of drinking soda pop. Remember, juice has its own natural sugars. There is a limit to how much juice that can be omitted in a day.

Pineapple Orange Yogurt Popsicles

3 ounces of frozen concentrated orange juice

3 ounces of frozen concentrated pineapple juice

1 pint of vanilla yogurt

1 ice tray

tooth picks

Alternative: paper cups

Alternative: popsicle sticks

Directions:

Mix the pineapple and orange juice and vanilla yogurt in a blender. Blend well. Pour into ice tray mixture and freeze. When slightly frozen place in middle of cubed mixture a tooth pick. Continue to freeze. Note: An alternative is to pour mixture into paper cups and freeze. When mixture is slightly frozen, place a popsicle stick in the middle of the cup and continue to let mixture freeze.

Mix Berries Parfait

1 tub of vanilla yogurt

1 cup of Raisin Bran Cereal or any generic

plastic parfait glass

Alternative: paper cups

non dairy whip topping

Mix together the following:

1 cup of fresh or frozen blueberries

1 cup of fresh or frozen raspberries

1 cup of fresh or frozen sliced strawberries

Directions:

Place on the bottom of parfait glass 1-1/2 tablespoons of fruit mixture. Then, place 2 tablespoons of yogurt on top of mixture. Repeat until mixture is 1/2 inch from the rim. Place 1 to 2 tablespoons of raisin bran in a zip lock bag and crush with hands. Sprinkle mixture on top. Place tablespoon of whip topping on top of raisin bran. Ready to Eat. Enjoy!!

Polar Ice Cubes

100% juice (any flavor)

glass of water

ice tray

Directions:

Pour juice into an ice tray and freeze thoroughly. In a glass of cool water place desired amount of cubes into the glass. This is great for summer hot summer days and for kids who don't like to drink water!

Taco Bagel Pizza

plain bagels

1 pound of cooked ground turkey

Alternative: cooked ground vegetarian burger meat

1cup of thick and chunky mild salsa

no fat cream cheese

8 ounce package of shredded taco blend cheese

Directions:

Brown turkey meat and drain. Mix one cup of salsa into turkey and simmer 5 to 10 minutes. Set aside. On each half bagel spread cream cheese evenly. Take one to two tablespoons of mcat mixture and sprinkle across bagel. Take shredded cheese and sprinkle a generous amount on top of meat. Place bagels on a cookie sheet and place in a preheated 350 degrees oven until cheese melts over pizza bagel. This usually takes 2 to 5 minutes. Make sure pizza bagel has cooled enough for little ones to handle. Enjoy! **Note:** You may use a toaster oven.

Veggie Croissant

1 large croissant

cucumbers, sliced

spinach leaves

bean sprouts

carrots, grated

tomatoes, thinly slice

White America Cheese

no fat or low fat mayo

Alternative: low fat salad dressing

mustard

golden raisins

Directions:

Cut croissant open without separating totally. Mix one tablespoon of mayo or salad dressing and one teaspoon of mustard and spread on both sides of croissant. Place cheese on croissant. Begin layers of vegetables with spinach leaves, then tomato slices, cucumber slices, bean sprouts, grated carrots. Sprinkle golden raisins on top. Cut into four pieces. Enjoy!!

Caribbean Island Fruit Sorbet

lime juice

lemon juice

½ cup of sugar

½ cup of water

1 cup of the following fruit pureed:

papaya, diced

kiwi, sliced

strawberries, diced (leave some whole)

3 small aluminum square pans

Directions:

Bring to a boil in a saucepan sugar and water. Let cool or refrigerate until ready to use. In a blender puree the kiwi and blend syrup mixture. Pour into a small square pan. Cover with plastic wrap and freeze. Break fruit into pieces and blend slightly until a smooth slush. Repeat process with 11/2 cup of diced papaya and 2 tablespoons of lime juice. Repeat process for 1 ½ cup of strawberries and 1 tablespoon of lemon juice. Serve in a parfait glass laying each fruit in the glass. Take a whole strawberry make a cut diagonal and place onto the rim of the glass for decoration.

Veggie Dip

½ cup of cottage cheese

½ cup of plain yogurt

1 package of powder ranch dressing mix

1 tablespoon of grated carrots

1 tablespoon of raisins

Directions:

Place in blender cottage cheese, yogurt and ranch mix. Blend well. Place mixture into a serving bowl and refrigerate until ready to use. Sprinkle raisins on top of mixture. Serve with veggies or spread over Ritz crackers. **Note:** Suggested vegetables are broccoli spears, celery sticks, carrot sticks, and cauliflower pieces.

Southern Fresh Rhubarb Strawberry Fruit Pie

½ cup of granulated sugar and brown sugar combined

1 tablespoon of cornstarch

¼ cup of enriched flour

4 cups of rhubarb, cut into ½ inch pieces

2 cups of thickly slice strawberries

1 tablespoon of orange juice

2 tablespoons of margarine or butter

1 teaspoon of ground nutmeg

Directions:

In bowl combine sugar mixture, cornstarch, flour nutmeg, rhubarb, strawberries and orange juice. Set aside. After completion of crust, place rhubarb mixture into crust, laying a top crust on mixture. Bake at 350 degree oven until fully cooked and crust is golden brown.

Directions for Pastry Crust:

2-1/4 cups of enrich flour,
salt
¾ cup of vegetable shortening

In a large bowl combine flour, salt and shortening. Blend together. Mead for two minutes. On a flour board, roll pastry dough out. Cut into round or square to fit the pan chosen.

Pineapple Sweet Potato

baked sweet potato

1 tablespoon of mini marshmallows

1 tablespoon of pineapple tidbits

1 teaspoon of brown sugar

1 pat of butter or margarine

½ teaspoon of cinnamon

½ teaspoon of nutmeg

Directions:

Place baked sweet potato on a plate. Cut open diagonal and spoon inside potato to make fluffy. Add butter or margarine, brown sugar, cinnamon and nutmeg. Blend in potato and fluff. Sprinkle on top marshmallows and pineapple. Serve **Note:** You can microwave the sweet potato for ten minutes turning every five during cooking process.

Trail Mix

1 cup of granola

½ cup of raisins

¼ cup of M&M Mini colored candy

¼ cup of almonds slices

¼ cup of dried cranberries

¼ cup of dried peaches or apricots

¼ cup of coconut flakes

Directions:

Mix ingredients in a large bowl, tossing to blend the mix. Place into ziploc bags to desired amount. Use for in between meals or snacks for **"On the Go"**. Serve with a glass of milk for beverage. Not intended for children under 3 years old.

Strawberry Cream Cheese Gingersnap Sandwich

12 to 16 ounces package of cream cheese

8 ounces of frozen strawberries

1 box of gingersnap wafers

Alternative: graham crackers

Directions:

Place into blender the cream cheese and blend on lowest speed. Slowly put in strawberries until mixture becomes thick and smooth, leaving some chunky pieces. Place into bowl and allow to set for 15 minutes. Spread generous amount on flat side of a gingersnap placing another wafer on top. Repeat

Cinnamon Spiced Applesauce

6 to 7 apples, peeled and diced

¼ cup of natural apple juice

1/3 cup of sugar

¼ teaspoon of cinnamon

raisins

Directions:

Place ingredients except for raisins into a bowl and microwave on high for 6 to 8 minutes. Put ingredients into blender or food processor until smooth texture. Place into serving bowls. Sprinkle raisins on top.

Peanut Butter Rice Crisp

4 tablespoon of butter or margarine

10 ounce package of marshmallows

6 cups of rice cereal

¼ cup of dried apple pieces

¼ cup of raisins

1 tablespoon of butter or margarine

Directions:

Place in a large bowl the rice cereal. Set aside. In a medium saucepan place in peanut butter, margarine or butter, marshmallows and melt over low heat. When melted remove from heat. With a wooden spoon pour mixture over rice cereal, coating cereal. Add dried apple pieces and raisins. Mix well. Place mixture into well greased pan and press mixture evenly into pan. Let cool at room temperature. Cut into squares. Enjoy!! **Note:** You may use almond butter in place of peanut butter. Instead of using stovetop, you may microwave on high until mixture is melted.

Turkey In A Bag

1 cup of shredded lettuce

1 cup of diced tomatoes

1 cup of shredded cheese

1 cup of diced black olives

1 cup of ground turkey meat

1 package of taco seasoning

1 tablespoon of sour cream

Individual serving of corn chips

Directions:

Brown ground turkey and drain off liquid. Mix in taco seasoning mix, following instructions on package. Set aside. Open corn chips making sure you don't tear the bag. Take 2 tablespoons of ground turkey and place into the corn chip bag. Take one handful of lettuce and place into bag. Take one tablespoon of each, black olives and tomatoes and place into bag. Shake well. Pour corn chip and meat mixture onto a plate. Sprinkle on top one tablespoon of shredded cheese. Top with a dab of sour cream. Upon completion, express it by saying, "Gobble, Gobble"!!

Friendship Fruit Salad

15 ounce can of tropical fruit (in its own juice)

15 ounce can of mandarin oranges

7 ounce package of coconut flakes

vanilla yogurt

sour cream

1 pound of bananas

Directions:

Place each ingredient into its own individual bowl. Make sure you cut the bananas into slices. Allow your child to pass each bowl to the person next to them starting on their right. After each person has taken a tablespoon of each ingredient and placed into their bowl, then blend together the ingredients. Then give your bowl to the person on your right until everyone has someone else's bowl.

Making Papa Bread

3 cups of grated carrots	¼ cup of vegetable oil
½ cup of butter or margarine	½ cup of raisins
½ cup of chopped walnuts or pecans	1 tablespoon of cinnamon
1 teaspoon of salt	½ teaspoon of nutmeg
1 tablespoon of baking powder	3 eggs
½ cup of milk	3 cups of enriched flour
½ cup of honey	½ cup of brown sugar

Directions:

Preheat oven to 350 degrees. Combine carrots, raisins, nuts, cinnamon, salt, nutmeg, baking powder, flour, sugar, honey. Mix well with electric beaters on lowest level. Add eggs, milk and margarine to mixture. Beat until mixture is well blended. Pour mixture into a well greased medium to large loaf pan. Bake at 350 degrees for 1 hour and 20 minutes or until knife inserted in the middle comes out clean. Serve with milk, fruit, cheese cubes or cheese sticks. Great snack with milk to leave out for that special someone during the holiday season.

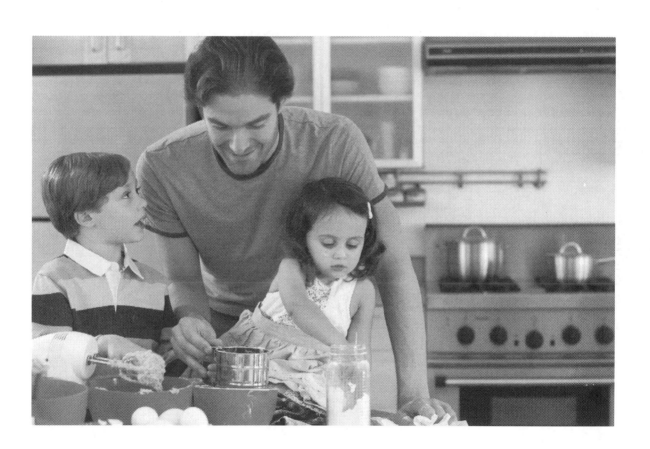

ACTIVITIES

How to Grow a Potato Plant

Each potato or potato piece only needs to have one small sprout to grow into a new potato plant. The pieces should weigh at least one and a half ounces with at least two or more sprout on it. For a garden dig a trench at least 6 inches deep in soil that has previously been tilled and fertilized. For a single plant place in a hole about four inches deep. Space plants twelve inches apart. Be careful not to break sprouts off from potato. Place the sprout upwards and cover sides with soil letting the top of the sprout show about six inches above soil. Mound soil around potato sprouts. As they grow continue to mound soil around until it gets twelve inches high.

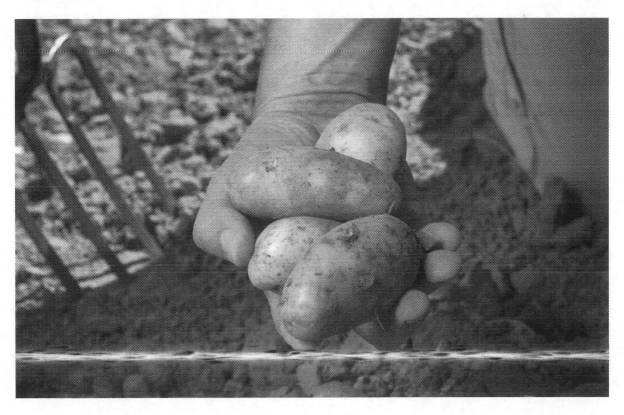

Where Do Vegetable Grow?

Began this activity with discussions of the following questions: Where do vegetables grow? Places where they may grow? Examples, under dirt or on a vine, on a tree? Discuss how some vegetables grow a flower first. Talk about farmers and what types of vegetables they grow in the U.S. What about farmers overseas? What types of vegetables do they grow? Read a book about farming. Sing "The Farmer and the Dell" and its circle game. Let each child take a turn at being the farmer who takes a wife or husband and choose others to be different animals on their farm. Examples are a cat, dog, goat, sheep, cow, duck, chicken, goose.

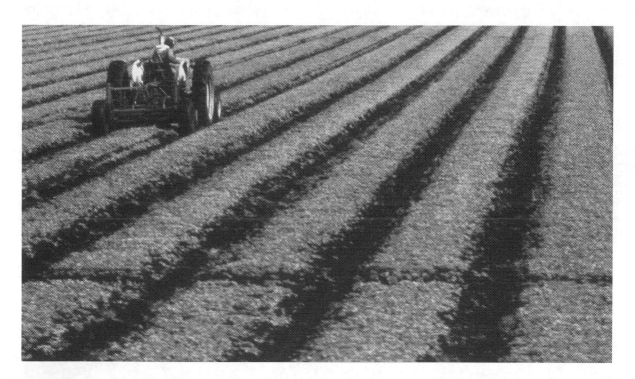

Multi Cultural Food "Hummus"

Discuss with your child how **"hummus"** is considered a main staple food n many countries. Israel made hummus a food symbol like the United States did with apple pie. In some countries such as in Arabia or Morocco, as a gesture of friendship, it is proper to sit on the floor on a rug and share from a bowl of hummus and pita bread with a shredded meat in gravy and vegetables. Try this tradition with your family. Place around the room flags of different countries that have hummus in their diet. Place a rug on the floor and serve your hummus, pita bread, meat and vegetables.

Making a Kooky Pineapple

Art supplies

10x5 cardboard

green feathers about an inch long

crayons or colored pencils

button eyes

glue

Draw a picture of a pineapple. Color your pineapple with yellow, gold blended into the pineapple. Use the brown color to make dots crisscross lines. Take the feathers and glue to the top of your pineapple for leaves. Glue on your button eyes onto your pineapple. Name your pineapple after you such as, "Bobby the Kooky Pineapple".

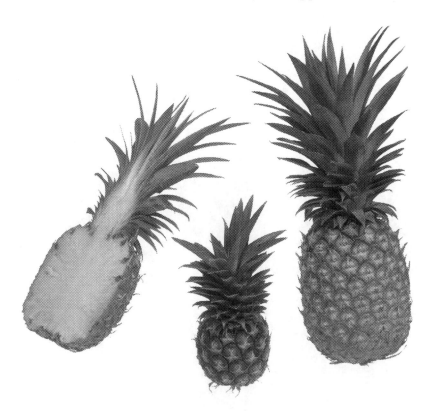

Celebrate Saint Patrick's Day

Drink:

Mix white grape juice with soda and add a drop of green food coloring.

Hat:

Art supplies

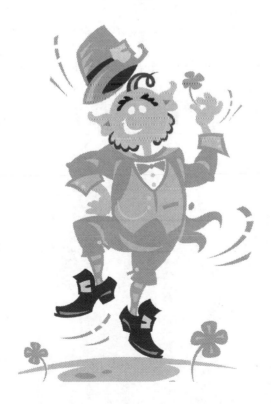

green tissue paper

scissors

glue

stapler

green card board paper

Snacks Can Be Nutritious And Good Choices For Kids

white card board paper

black card board paper

gold glitter

Directions: Measure your child's head around giving about an extra inch or two. For height of hat measure about ten inches. Cut two pieces of the white card board to the fruit measurements of your child's head length and ten inches for width. Staple the two ends pieces together of one cardboard so that it fits on top of the child's head. Cut a round piece of card board to fit on top to seal hat close. Take the other piece of cardboard and fold about one inch on length. Unfold and wrap folded end around the bottom of hat gluing it into place. This will serve as the brim of the hat. You may staple the back close to secure. Let dry. Take green tissue paper and begin to glue onto hat any way you wish as long as the hat is completely covered and the brim. Remember, make sure the under side of brim is cover with the tissue paper also. Allow to dry for ten minutes. Cut a piece of the black card board to the measurement of your child's head. Take the black piece and glue it around the bottom of the hat next to the brim. Cut a small square piece of the white card board to resemble a belt buckle. Fold square and cut out of the middle another square. Squeeze and spread glue on one side of square. Sprinkle gold glitter onto square covering area. Shake lose glitter that did not stick. Spread glue onto other side of square and press onto black card board in middle in front on the hat. Let dry. Happy Saint Patrick's Day!!

Ice Cream Day

Activity: Celebrate Ice Cream Day! Talk about how ice cream is made and what their

favorite flavor. Discuss how in older days there were little boys who pushed ice cream carts. Example; the similarity of paperboys which had a route in a neighborhood, so did the ice cream boys to make extra money. Explain how we have ice cream trucks today that come into different neighborhoods. If you grew up in this era or know stories from your parents, share the stories with your children. What was your favorite ice cream from the ice cream boy? Here is a word puzzle to find words connected to ice cream.

I	B	U	B	B	L	E	G	U	M	P	Q	Y
D	C	F	Y	R	R	E	B	W	A	R	T	S
L	H	E	I	E	L	P	P	A	E	N	I	P
E	E	G	J	C	H	O	C	O	L	A	T	E
M	R	K	U	V	R	A	I	N	B	O	W	N
R	R	Z	T	U	N	R	E	T	T	U	B	O
A	Y	V	A	N	I	L	L	A	T	R	A	C
C	D	N	O	M	L	A	T	N	I	M	K	H

List of Words

Cherry	Cone
Bubble Gum	Mint Almond
Vanilla	Cart
Chocolate	Pineapple
Strawberry	Butternut
Rainbow	Carmel

Beach Day

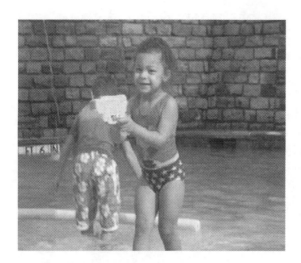
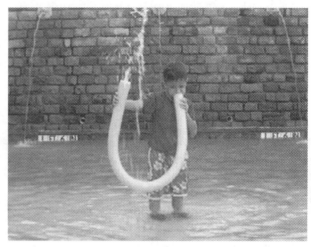

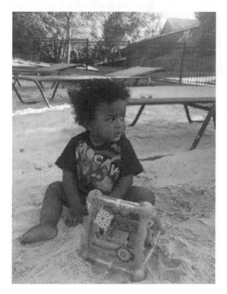

Today is a great day to go to the beach! One way to celebrate is to go to the pool and pretend that you're at the beach. Kids have great imagination. If a pool is a not available there are other ways to celebrate "Beach Day". Have a sandbox? If not you can lay a piece of heavy plastic on the ground outdoors and pour sand on it. Get a couple of beach towels, noodles, water guns, lounge folding chairs or beach chairs, put on your bathing suit and wear your best beach hat. Kids love to run through the sprinkler system. Be creative and think of other ways to celebrate "Beach day".

Friends

Talk with your child about friendship. Ask them what they think a friend is? What is the difference between a friend and a best friend? What do best friends do together? Do they share? Do they play games together? Do you tell your secrets to them that no one else knows? Can a friend be an animal like your dog or cat? Can your best friend be your mom or dad? Ask them can you make new friends? You will be surprise at some of the answers you will get. There was an old television series that aired years ago called, "The Courtship of Eddie's Father". The theme song was "Let Me Tell You About My Best Friend" which happened to be his father. Play songs about a person being your best friend or read stories or even show a movie about best friends. Most children television channels have stories and videos on subjects of being friends. Try your community library to get a book or a video.

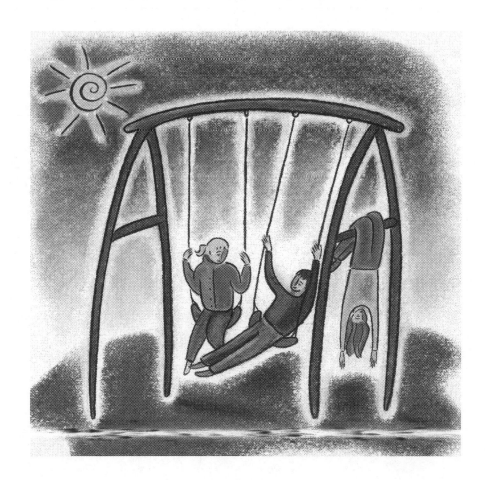

Picture Book

Art Supplies

<u>All felt sheets are 5x7</u>	Single hole	puncher fun foam
2 blue square felt sheets	Dark green ribbon	cookie cutter
2 red square felt sheets	Dark blue ribbon	small peel and spell letters
2 green square felt sheets	4 card board squares	
2 yellow square felt sheets	Button eyes	
glue	6 Photo Holders (cardboard or foam)	*Note:* You may buy precut shapes

Directions:

Take card boards and glue felt squares on top of each side of the cardboards front and back. Alternate colors. Glue photo holders onto middle of felt cardboards on back of front cover and front of back cover. Glue on both sides for the rest of the cardboards. Allow to dry fully. For front cover cut a shape out of fun foam using a cookie cutter. The cookie cutter for example for a boy a red train or blue sail boat. For a girl, a pink teddy bear or a a big yellow bow. There are other pre-cut shapes available at your craft store. Glue a shape to the front of cover picture book and onto the back side of your last cardboard. Glue button eyes on front cover and use peel and stick to spell their names. Take hole puncher a and punch 2 holes on each left side of cardboard. Secure picture book with ribbon

Polar Snowman

Art Supplies

1 large white form ball	3 whole cloves	silver glitter
1 medium white form ball	2 tooth picks	cotton balls
1 small white form ball	1 small thimble	
1 ½ inch of black/red/green ribbon	3 small green buttons	
1 bottle of glue	small wooden square	

Directions

Glue medium ball onto large one. Then glue the small ball onto the medium ball. You may have to wait until one dries before gluing the other. Glue thimble on top of the small ball as the snowman's hat. Let dry. Cut ribbon to resemble a scarf. Place a small amount of glue in the middle of ribbon and place around the snowman between the small and medium ball. You may have to place a small amount to front to make scarf lay down. On middle of ball glue the 3 buttons. Take left over ribbon cut out 2 mittens and glue to tooth picks. Push tooth picks as arms into each side of snowman of middle ball. Push cloves for eyes and nose on the small ball. Glue snowman to wooden square. Spread a little glue on square around snowman and place cotton balls on top. Squeeze a little glue on top of cotton balls and sprinkle glitter on top. Carefully shake off loose glitter. Allow to dry over night.

Cinco De Mayo Kite

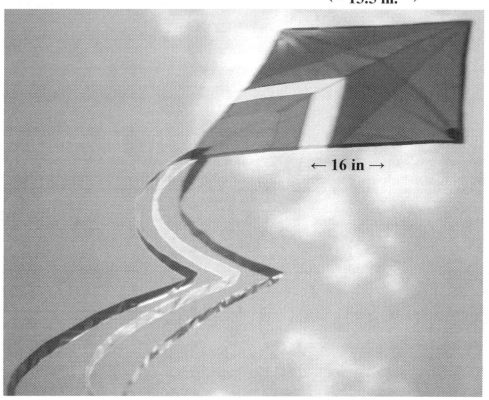

Art Supplies

Cookie cutters	various colors of fun foam
(2) 30 inch thick plastic sticks	ball of kite string
18 inches of ribbon	2 small jingle bells

Directions

Cut a piece of fun foam to the measurements of triangle in above illustration. With a single hole puncher; punch a hole in the middle of the kite and each ends of your kite. You should be at least ½ to 1 inch from the edge. Let your child cut different shapes from different colors of fun foam. To make different shapes use various cookie cutters of letters (to spell their name), animals, trees, or geometric shapes. Glue shapes to kite. Allow to fully dry to secure where shapes will not come off. Cut sticks to length of kite vertical and horizontal. At each end carve a groove so that the ends will slide over fun foam in place through hole punch at ends and crossing over one another as a "**t**". At bottom end of kite tie ribbon onto stick and slide other end through hole to front side of kite. Take jiggle bells and slide onto ribbon and tie knot to secure placing distance between them. Turn over kite and secure middle with kite string, wrapping it several times. **Happy Cinco De Mayo!!**

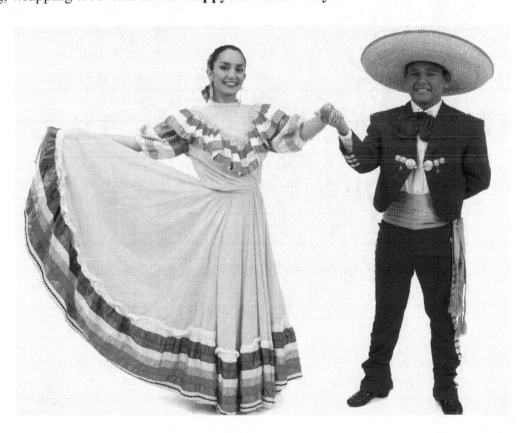

Making a Pot of Roses

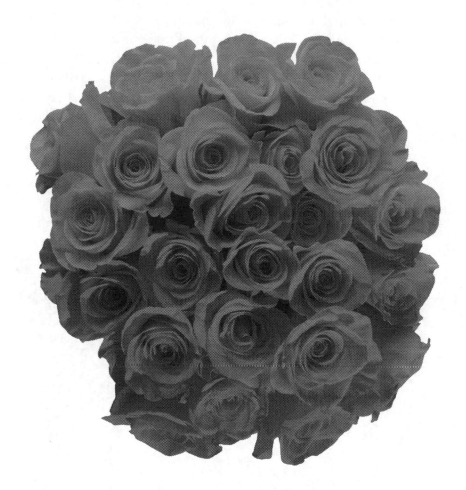

6" diameter styrofoam ball
4 types of felt (red, yellow, and pink, white, orange)
hot glue gun with glue sticks
flower pot (clay or plastic)

Small bag of moss
flora tape
flower wooden spikes

Note: Pot opening should be smaller than the diameter of your ball

Directions:

To make flowers; first pencil onto felt an outline of a three to four leaf clover. Make one clover small, one medium (a little bigger than the small one), then the last one larger than the medium one. Place one on top of the other; starting with the larger one making the clovers appear un- level from the other one. Push your finger in the middle on top the pinch them together at the middle of the bottom one. Then push together to get flower effect and or if petal look is not seen after pushing together, fold to get petal look. Take a spike and place at fold. Then take flora tape and begin to wrap around flower and spike until secure. Repeat for other flowers. Note: For added protection glue before taping. You may make the flowers any size you choose. Place styrofoam ball into pot. Stream hot glue onto top of ball and spread moss on top. Begin to arrange flowers into your pot.

On the Animal Trail

Activity

This is a great chance to take your children to the zoo!! See the excitement of your children as they learn about animals like the lion, the elephant and the giraffe. Read a book about the different animals they will see at the zoo and what the animals eat before you take your trip. Pack a lunch for the trip or bring your favorite trail mix. Pretend you're an animal at the zoo and make wild animal sounds and movements. If you're not able to go to the zoo, take a hike on a wooded trail in the park and pretend they are wild animals moving about. Of course you may see a skunk, a squirrel or a raccoon but it's the excitement of pretending. Allow the children to even draw a picture of their favorite zoo animal. Hang it proudly on the wall or refrigerator. Happy Trails!!

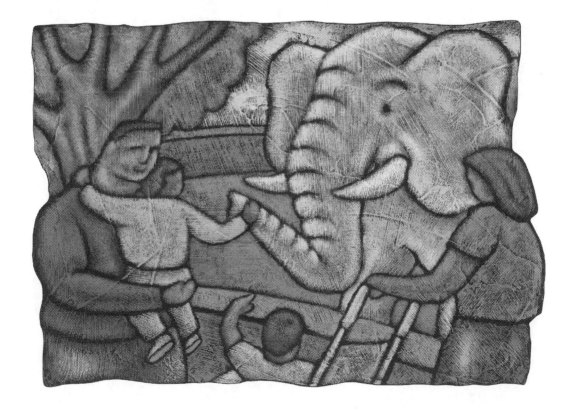

Johnny Apple Seed

Opportunity knocks especially during the Fall months to go to the apple farm. Your child will enjoy going to the farm to pick apples, take a hay ride on the back of the wagon as you ride the trail to see the change of the Fall leaves colors while drinking hot apple cider. Read the story about **"Johnny Apple Seed"** before you go to the farm. There are many activities offered at most apple farms. Make your favorite apple snack with the apples you picked from the farm and or play the game of "Dunking for Apples". While there make it a memory and take a picture of the occasion.

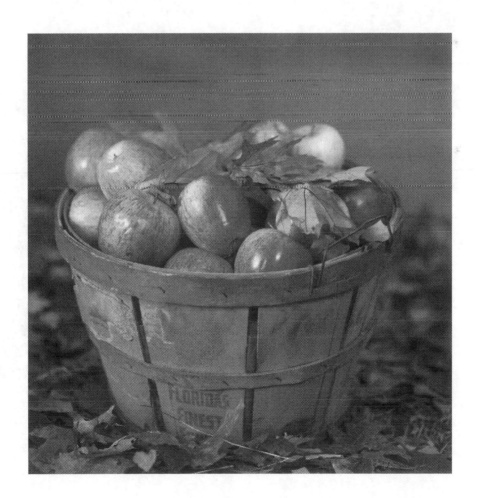

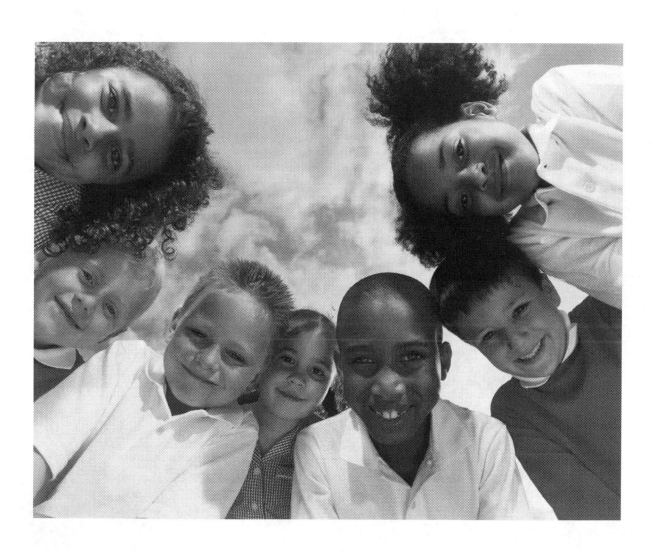

EXTRAS

Food Record

Time	Food	Beverage	Amount	Hunger	Mood	Others

Child's Serving Size

Breakfast	1-2 Years	3-5 Years	6-12 Years
Food Group			
Milk	½ cup	¾ cup	1 cup
!00% Juice Fruit or Vegetable	¼ cup	½ cup	½ cup
Grains or Breads	½ slice	½ slice	1 slice
Cold Cereals	¼ cup	¼ cup	½ cup
Hot Cereals	¼ cup	¼ cup	½ cup
Snacks			
Select only two of the following:			
Milk	½ cup	½ cup	1 cup
100% Juice Fruit or Vegetable	½ cup	½ cup	¾ cup
Grains or Breads	½ slice	½ slice	1 slice
Meats or Meat Alternative	½ ounce	½ ounce	1 ounce
Yogurt	¼ cup or 2 oz.	¼ cup or 2 oz.	½ cup or 4 oz.
Lunch/Supper			
Milk	½ cup	¾ cup	1 cup
Vegetables or fruit (2 or more)	¼ cup	½ cup	¾ cup
Grains/Breads	½ slice	½ slice	1 slice
Meat or poultry or Fish	1 ounce	1 ½ ounce	2 ounces
Cheese	1 ounce	1 ½ ounce	2 ounces
Cottage Cheese	¼ cup or 2 oz.	3/8 cup or 3 oz.	½ cup or 4 oz.
Eggs	½ egg	¾ egg	1 egg
Cooked Dry Beans or Peas	¼ cup	3/8 cup	½ cup

Snacks Can Be Nutritious And Good Choices For Kids

Peanut Butter, soy Butter, Almond Butter	2 tablespoons	3 tablespoons	4 tablespoons
Peanuts, Soy nuts, Tree Nuts or Seeds	½ ounce	¾ ounce	1 ounce
Yogurt	½ cup or 4 oz.	¾ cup or 6 oz.	1 cup or 8 oz.

Fiber Rich Foods

Vitamin C

Asparagus	Okra	Grapefruit Juice 100%
Broccoli	Potatoes	Honey Dew Melon
Brussels Sprouts	Peas	Oranges
Cabbage	Rutabagas	Orange Juice100%
Cauliflower	Tomatoes	Raspberries
Green Beans	Tomato Juice 100%	Strawberries
Green Leafy Vegetables (Greens)	Turnips	Tangelos
Green Bell Peppers	Cantaloupe	Tangerines
Lima Beans	Grapefruit	Watermelon

Vitamin A

Asparagus	Peas	Apricots
Broccoli	Pumpkin	Cantaloupe
Carrots	Sweet Potatoes or Yams	Cherries
Green leafy Vegetables (greens)	Spinach	Nectarines
Kale	Tomatoes	Peaches
Mix Vegetables	Tomato Juice 100%	Plums/Prunes

Iron Rich Foods

Vegetables	Fruits	Meats	Meat Alternatives	Grains	Combination Foods	Milk
Artichoke	Bananas	Eggs	Almonds	Bran Flakes	Beef & Bean Burrito	Soy
Collard Greens	Cranberries	Ham	Baked Beans	Bran Muffins, Waffles & Tortilla	Chili W Beans or Meat	Soy Butter
Green Beans	Raisins	Liver	Black Beans	Corn Flakes	French Toast	
Mixed Vegetables	Dried Prunes	Oysters	Dried Beans/ Peas and Vegetarian Beans	Enriched Cereals w/45% Iron	Lasagna w/ Meat	
Black-eyed Peas	Prune Juice 100%	Shrimp	Lima Beans	Granola W/ Raisins	Macaroni and Cheese	
Green Peas	Strawberries	Turkey	Refried Beans	Rice	Marinara Sauce w/Meat	
Spinach	Watermelon	Tuna	Peanut, Soy & Almond Butter	Oatmeal	Pizza W/ Cheese or meat	
Tomato Juice			Hummus Dip	Enriched Pastas	Taco w/Meat and Cheese	
			Sunflower Seeds		Vegetable Soup	
			Walnuts		Vegetable Beef Stew	

Buying Calendar for Fresh Fruits Usually Found In Stores

January	February	March
Apples Avocados Grapefruit Tangerines Navel Oranges Lemons Pears	Apples Avocados Grapefruit Lemons Navel Oranges Tangerines Pears	Apples Avocados Grapefruit Lemons Navel Oranges Tangerines Pears

Snacks Can Be Nutritious And Good Choices For Kids

April	May	June
Apples Avocados Grapefruit Lemons Navel Oranges Strawberries Pears	Avocados Cherries Grapefruit Lemons Navel Oranges Pears Valencia Oranges	Apricots Avocados Blueberries Cantaloupe Cherries Figs Honeydew Melons Lemons Nectarines Peaches Plums Strawberries Valencia Oranges Watermelon
July	**August**	**September**
Apricots Avocados Blueberries Cantaloupe Grapefruit Lemons Honeydew Melons Pears Nectarines Plums Strawberries Peaches Valencia Oranges Watermelon	Avocados Cantaloupes Figs Grapes Grapefruit Lemons Honeydew Melons Nectarines Valencia Oranges Peaches Plums Watermelon Pears	Apples Cantaloupe Figs Honeydew Melons Grapefruit Grapes Lemons Peaches Pears Plums Prunes
October	**November**	**December**
Apples Dates Figs Grapes Lemons Pears Persimmons Valencia Oranges	Apples Avocados Dates Grapes Lemons Persimmons	Apples Avocados Dates Grapefruit Lemons Navel Oranges
Note: Walnuts are available in November and December		

Buying Calendar for Vegetables Usually Found In Stores

January	February	March
Beets Cabbage Cauliflower Celery Lettuce Potatoes Spinach	Artichokes Asparagus Beets Cabbage Celery Lettuce Potatoes Spinach	Artichokes Asparagus Beets Broccoli Cabbage Carrots Cauliflower Celery Potatoes

Snacks Can Be Nutritious And Good Choices For Kids

April	May	June
Artichokes Asparagus Beets Broccoli Carrots Cauliflower Lettuce Peas Spinach	Asparagus Beets Cabbage Carrots Celery Lettuce Onions Peas Potatoes Spinach Corn Tomatoes	Carrots Celery Cucumbers Onions Green Snap Beans Lettuce Peppers Potatoes Squash Corn Tomatoes
July	**August**	**September**
Cabbage Carrots Beets Broccoli Celery Cucumbers Eggplant Green Snap Beans Lettuce Green Lima Beans Okra Onions Peppers Potatoes Squash Corn Tomatoes	Cabbage Celery Cucumbers Eggplant Lettuce Okra Onions Peppers Potatoes Squash Corn Tomatoes Green Snap Beans	Cabbage Cucumbers Eggplant Green Snap Beans Onions Peas Peppers Squash Corn
October	**November**	**December**
Broccoli Brussels Sprouts Cabbage Cucumbers Eggplant Green Beans Lima Beans Lettuce Okra Peas Peppers Potatoes Corn Sweet Potatoes Tomatoes Winter Squash	Broccoli Brussels Sprouts Lettuce	Broccoli Brussels Sprouts Carrots Cauliflower Celery Potatoes Spinach Sweet Potatoes

Eight Ways to Move

Physical exercise is a part of everyday life that can keep you fit and healthy. Everyone have certain levels of exercise activity they can accomplish. You can do some movements to increase your activity level in order to improve your health. Physicians recommend at least 30 minutes of exercise sessions per day will help in improving your overall physical health. Here are some easy ways to get yourself or your children started.

- ♥ Go on a 15-30 minute walk with the children. Note: If you have an infant use the stroller
- ♥ Ride your bikes
- ♥ Go roller skating with the children
- ♥ Play a game such as "kick ball"
- ♥ Play volleyball
- ♥ Go swimming
- ♥ Turn the music on and dance
- ♥ Have a contest to see who can do the most sit-ups, push-ups, jumping jacks or runs the fastest.

Remember, children love to have play time and when the parents join in, it becomes more exciting and challenging. This will help your children and you to bond, and to get a better night's sleep, and also improves your health.

Playing For Exercise

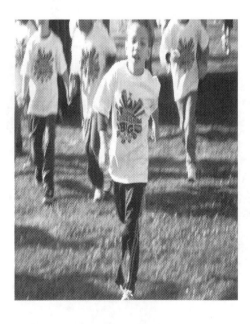
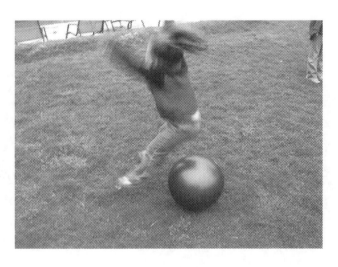

Truths

1. Cutting out all starches such as breads, pasta and potatoes will help me to lose weight. **True or False**

   Answer: False. Carbohydrates are low in fat and a great source of energy. Foods such as butter, cream sauces, regular sour cream causes extra Calories to an otherwise great food.

2. If you buy frozen or canned vegetables, you are missing out on important vitamins and minerals. **True or False**

   Answer: False. Vegetables that have been frozen or canned immediately after they are harvest may be more nutrient dense than many fresh vegetables. Frozen and canned vegetables are convenient and nutritious.

3. Lean meat can be lower in fat than poultry. **True or False**

   Answer: True. Poultry with skin and if its fried has more fat than lean cuts of meat. Three ounces of baked chicken with skin has thirteen grams of fat compared to three ounces of beef round or pork tenderloin which has only four grams of fat.

4. Jogging two miles burns more calories than walking two miles. **True or False**

   Answer: False. They are approximately the same amount of calories in either activity. The difference is the amount of time it takes to complete two miles.

5. "Eat Five a Day" What does it mean?
   - A.   Eat a food from all five food groups daily.
   - B.   Eat five servings of bread, pasta, rice or other grains daily.
   - C.   Eat at least five fruits and vegetables servings daily
   - D.   Eat three meals plus two snacks daily.

   Answer: C. According to the advice of nutrition experts and the Daily Guide Pyramid, we should strive to eat at least 3 servings of vegetables and at least 2 servings of fruit per day. The Food Guide Pyramid suggests the amount of vegetables should be between 3-5 servings and the amount of fruit should be at least 2-4 servings.

6. Which fruits and vegetables provide the most nutrients of vitamin A, vitamin C, source of folate and potassium? Below is a list of fruits and vegetables. Match the nutrient to the list below. Answers on page 53.

Lists	1	2	3	4
	carrots	kiwi	orange juice	sweet potato
	spinach	broccoli	romaine lettuce	bananas
	mango	turnip greens	green peas	apricots
	tomatoes	cantaloupe	peanuts	baked beans

Foods to Keep With You For "On The Go Snacks

Whole Wheat Crackers   100% Fruit Juice Box

Bottle Water   Carrot Sticks

Celery Sticks   Box of Raisins

Graham Crackers   Trail Mix (see recipe)

Peanut Butter

<u>Fresh Fruits</u>

Apples	Bananas	Grapes	Peaches
Kiwi	Oranges	Strawberries	Plums

There are pre-packages foods that are nutritious for snacks for "On The Go" such as the following:

Peanut Butter Crackers (whole wheat)

Cheese Crackers (whole wheat)

Box of Fruit Snacks (100%)

Kitchen Fun!!

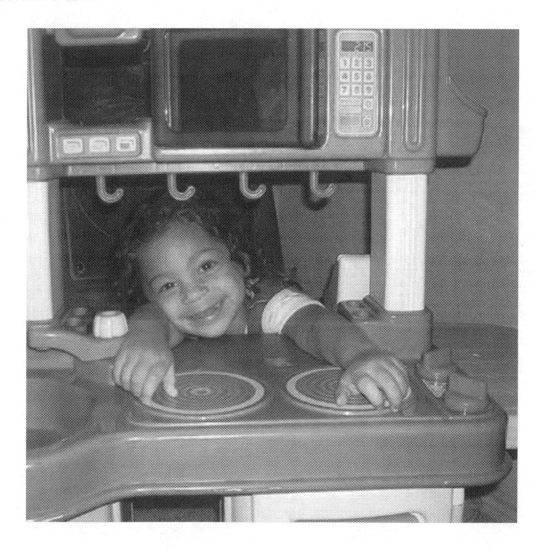

Additional Sources for Health and Nutrition

Food and Nutrition Information Center
National Agricultural Library, USDA
1301 Baltimore Blvd. Room 304
Beltsville MD. 20705-2351

United States Dept of Agricultural
Fruit and Vegetable Market News
www.usda.gov

The American Dietetic Association
www.eatright.org

The American Red Cross
http://www.redcross.org

United States Health and Human Services
200 Independence Avenue, S.W.
Washington, D.C. 20201
www.hhs.gov

The American Heart Association
7272 Greenville Ave.
Dallas, TX 75231
(888) 242-2453 (Inside U.S.)
(214) 570-5935 (Outside U.S.)
8 a.m.—5 p.m. M-F CDT (USA)
www.heart.org,

The Diabetes Institute
1701 North Beauregard Street
Alexandria, VA 22311
1-800-DIABETES (800-342-2383)
www.diabetes.org

The United Way
http://liveunited.org

Local Area:
State of . . . .
Health and Human Services Commission
TANF/Food Stamps
Nutrition Education Training

Page 50
Answers to question 6 1. Vitamin A, 2. Vitamin C, 3. Foliate, 4. Potassium

Good Morning Bright Eyes!!

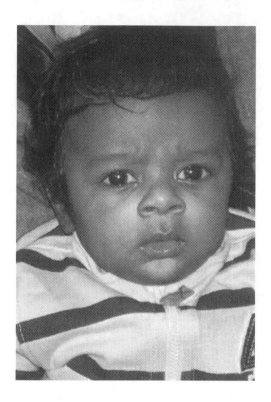

Playground Fun!!

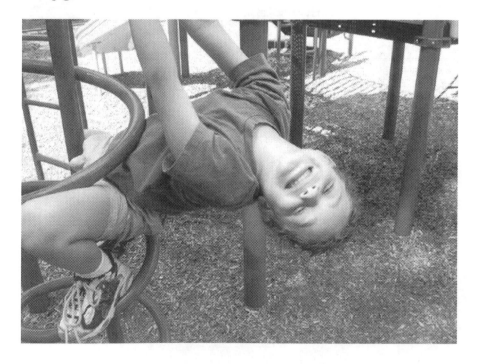